YOUR KNOWLEDGE HAS VALUE

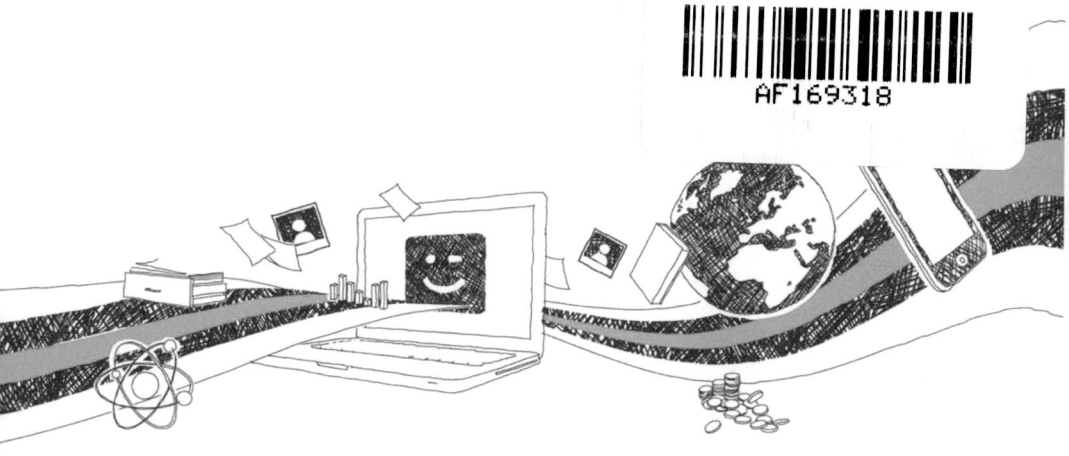

- We will publish your bachelor's and master's thesis, essays and papers

- Your own eBook and book - sold worldwide in all relevant shops

- Earn money with each sale

Upload your text at www.GRIN.com
and publish for free

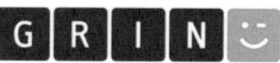

Bibliographic information published by the German National Library:

The German National Library lists this publication in the National Bibliography; detailed bibliographic data are available on the Internet at http://dnb.dnb.de .

This book is copyright material and must not be copied, reproduced, transferred, distributed, leased, licensed or publicly performed or used in any way except as specifically permitted in writing by the publishers, as allowed under the terms and conditions under which it was purchased or as strictly permitted by applicable copyright law. Any unauthorized distribution or use of this text may be a direct infringement of the author s and publisher s rights and those responsible may be liable in law accordingly.

Imprint:

Copyright © 2018 GRIN Verlag
Print and binding: Books on Demand GmbH, Norderstedt Germany
ISBN: 9783668682252

This book at GRIN:

https://www.grin.com/document/419464

Patrick Kimuyu

The Role of Behavioral and Cognitive Theory in Phobia Development and Extinction

GRIN Verlag

GRIN - Your knowledge has value

Since its foundation in 1998, GRIN has specialized in publishing academic texts by students, college teachers and other academics as e-book and printed book. The website www.grin.com is an ideal platform for presenting term papers, final papers, scientific essays, dissertations and specialist books.

Visit us on the internet:

http://www.grin.com/

http://www.facebook.com/grincom

http://www.twitter.com/grin_com

The Role of Behavioral and Cognitive Theory in Phobia Development and Extinction

Name: Patrick Kimuyu

Table of Contents

Introduction 3

Case Study Overview 3

    Describing Sally's Phobia Using Inference and Research of the Development of Simple Phobias 4

Explaining Phobia through Behavioral and Cognitive Theory 5

    Classical conditioning 5

    Operant conditioning 6

    Observational learning 7

The Process of Extinction in Overcoming Phobia 7

Tenets of Cognitive Theory in Overcoming Phobia 8

Conclusion 9

References 10

Introduction

Phobia is increasingly becoming a central point of attraction in the field of emotion research. Research psychologists are interested in generating more evidence to reconcile the wide differences that exist from the current findings. From a critical perspective, consensus on the basis of fear or phobia appears to be unlikely in the foreseeable future. This is attributable to the fact that psychologists perceive phobia as a psychological construct, whereas biologists argue fear to be an aspect that is discoverable through scientific inquiry. Another aspect that has contributed to the controversy surrounding research on phobia is the lack of consensus on how to investigate this emotion. Despite these controversies, clinical scientists are still engaged in intensive research on fear as an underlying aspect in mood and anxiety disorders. From a real-life perspective, phobias are not new in animals, including humans. As such, Adolphs (2013) perceives fear to be a central state of organisms. This case study report provides a comprehensive discussion based on the psychological construction of emotions through the application of behavioral and cognitive theory in analyzing the given case study.

Case Study Overview

The case study involves Sally, a 23-year-old woman who is reported to have developed dog phobia during her childhood. She is said to have had negative experience with dogs, as an aspect that is apparently the cause of her dog phobia. Surprisingly, her phobia seems to be causing anxiety in her, interfering with the way she interacts with other people during day-to-day social interactions. Her dog phobia has filled her life with anxiety; she is always anxious whenever she meets new people or invited to unfamiliar areas.

Overall, Sally's fear for dogs provides an opportunity to explore a number of aspects that are associated with phobias. Foremost, it offers an opportunity to discuss the potential ways for the development of simple phobias. It also offers an opportunity to discuss how extinction and cognitive learning are useful psychological tools for helping people to recover from their phobias.

Describing Sally's Phobia Using Inference and Research of the Development of Simple Phobias

Sally's phobia can be described from the perspective of how simple phobias, including dog phobia develops. In this context, this behavior can be explained through an analytical review of the underlying relationship between emotion and cognition. This way, it is possible to trace the process involved in the development of simple phobias. Specifically, information processing theories explain the cognitive process and its cognitive products. In retrospect, it is apparent that behavioral theory of anxiety has generated an immense impact on information processing approaches to emotion due to its reliance on the conditioning model. This perspective explains how anxiety is acquired and maintained within an individual. For the case of Sally, she acquired dog phobia as a result of negative experience she encountered while in her childhood. Since then, she has not been able to shed off fear of dogs. Instead, this form of anxiety has remained to her early adulthood, and this can be explained by theories of acquisition and maintenance of this disorder. In other words, Sally's dog phobia falls under the two-process theory that holds the assumption that conditioning underpins the fixing of behaviors; thus, active counter-conditioning interventions are required to change these behaviors. However, a different dimension exists in cognitive psychology that seeks to address clinical problems. This approach holds that emotional responses can be changed through the alteration of events or meaning associated to the underlying events. This approach focuses on investigating specific beliefs that are responsible for dysfunctional patterns of cognitive processes and replaces them with beneficial beliefs (Crocker et al., 2013). Based on this, inferences can be made on how simple phobias develop. Evidence shows that fear structures influence attentional strategies and this leads to behavioral and cognitive avoidance (Foa & Kozak, 1986). It is reported that fear structure involves an encounter of a stimuli from the environment which leads to the formation of networks in memory. Consequently, the interaction between emotion and memory generates mechanisms to escape the danger associated with the stimuli through the activation of the escape sequence. This way, an individual develops propositional meaning to the stimuli. As a result, he is able to discriminate non-threat situations from threat situations (Krypotos, Effting, Kindt & Beckers, 2015). In the case for Sally, the negative experience she acquired in second grade was the stimuli that triggered fear responses as it is evidenced by her behavior of avoiding dogs. This implies that phobic anxiety has profound effects on memory.

Explaining Phobia through Behavioral and Cognitive Theory

In retrospect, phobia can be explained extensively by three main approaches; classical conditioning, operant conditioning and observational learning. These are the main ways through which abnormal behavior can be formed. From a behavioral approach, operant conditioning, classical conditioning and social learning theory have been used to explain the occurrence of several psychological disorders, including phobias (Henton & Iversen, 2012).

Classical conditioning

From the perspective of classical conditioning, it is argued that associative learning and classical conditioning underlie the development of phobias. In this context, it is possible to deduce individual's association with stimuli that trigger anxiety through classical conditioning. This approach is based on the tenets of behaviorism which hold that environment plays an integral role in shaping behavior. They also posit that learning occurs as a result of interactions with the environment. Overall, classical conditioning entails the formation of an association between two stimuli. This association is believed to result to a learned response.

Classical conditioning occurs in three main phases. The first phase occurs before conditioning through which a naturally occurring stimulus triggers a response. This is referred to as unconditioned stimulus (UCS) and its resultant response is referred to as unconditioned response (UCR). An outstanding example of scenario is when someone encounters the smell of food. This unconditioned stimulus triggers stimulus, which in this case is an unconditioned response. At the same time when the unconditioned stimulus occurs, a neutral stimulus occurs, as well, which is not associated with any response. The second phase of classical conditioning involves the pairing of the unconditioned stimulus with the neutral stimulus leading to the development of an association between these stimuli. At this point the neutral stimulus is transformed into a conditioned stimulus (CS) (Henton & Iversen, 2012). This is referred to as the conditioning process which involves the conditioning of the neutral stimulus as a result of its association with the unconditioned stimulus. Finally, the third phase occurs after conditioning through which a learned response or a conditioned response is expressed through behavior. For the case of Sally, avoidance of dogs was a conditioned response.

Operant conditioning

Phobia can also be explained by operant conditioning. Unlike, classical conditioning that explains the development of phobias, operant conditioning advances a step further to explain why phobias are maintained. In other words, it explains the underlying forces which reinforce the existence of phobias; thus, inhibiting their decay over time (Henton & Iversen, 2012). Overall, operant conditioning is believed to be responsible for maintaining phobia.

Operant conditioning holds that phobias are maintained through negative reinforcement. It is believed that removal of an unpleasant consequence strengthens avoidance behavior

(Doctor, Kahn & Adamec, 2010). The case of Sally serves as an outstanding example. Sally is said to have dog phobia so every time she sees a dog she tries to avoid it. She even avoids places with dogs. This way, Sally's avoidance of dogs reduces her feelings of anxiety. As she tries to reduce her anxiety, she negatively reinforces her behavior of avoiding dogs; thus, maintaining her dog phobia. This is the same case with everyone who has phobia, avoidance negatively reinforces the resultant behavior and maintains phobia.

Observational learning

In reality, animals attempt to learn on how to respond to environmental stimuli that pose a threat to their survival. This explains why animals, including humans develop adaptive mechanisms to resist the adverse effects of environmental stimuli. Observational (social) learning theory holds that animals are able to learn thro7ugh observing actions of another animal, or through interaction (Galef, 1988). According to Fryling, Johnston, and Hayes (2011), observational learning approach implies that observation may lead to behavioral change. From a critical perspective, three experiences emerge from the learning theory: stimulus; stimulus-stimulus; and response-reinforcement. The first experience may involve a verbal command, whereas the second and the third involve paired events. For instance, Sally's dog phobia is reported to have been caused by negative experiences she had with dogs during her childhood. It might have been that her encounters with dogs were accompanied by attacks. This could have been a stimulus-stimulus experience.

The Process of Extinction in Overcoming Phobia

In practice, the process of extinction plays integral roles in overcoming phobias. Evidence indicates that reducing CS-US expectancy reduces conditioned responses (Lipp & Edwards, 2002). Further evidence reveals that changes in contingency beliefs and expectancies can be stored in long-term memory, and helps in extinction of phobias (Hofmann, 2008). In classical conditioning, extinction of a phobia is associated with the disappearance of pairing between an unconditional stimulus and the conditional stimulus, leading to the decrease or disappearance of the conditioned response. For the case of Sally, the process of extinction can be applied to overcome her phobia in several ways. First, if seeing dogs (the unconditional stimulus) accompanied by barking (the conditional stimulus) is what causes panic, she can be exposed to one of these stimuli while the other stimulus is controlled. This way, the pairing between the unconditional stimulus and the conditional stimulus will be eliminated leading to the disappearance of the conditioned response (dog avoidance).

Tenets of Cognitive Theory in Overcoming Phobia

From a professional perspective, the tenets of cognitive theory can be used to help Sally overcome her phobia. This can be done through cognitive restructuring (Beard, 2011). In this context, a therapist can interview Sally to identify the 'self-talk' of what goes on in Sally's head whenever she encounters dogs. This can be followed by a focused analysis to test if what Sally thinks about dogs is actually true or false. Alternatively, Sally's phobia can be approached from cognitive biases: attention bias and interpretation bias. She can be helped to develop positive signals towards dogs to replace the negative ones (Seligman & Ollendick, 2011).

Conclusion

Conclusively, phobias develop through classical conditioning and observational learning. Classical conditioning enhances the development of phobia through the interaction of the unconditional and neutral stimuli which, in turn produce the conditional stimuli that leads to the conditional response. On the other hand, operant conditioning helps in maintaining phobia through negative reinforcement. Cognitive restructuring can help in treating phobia. In practice, cognitive theory has been applied in the treatment of anxiety disorders including phobia. Therefore, Sally's dog phobia can be addressed through masking one of the stimuli, either the neutral or the unconditional stimulus. This will lead to the disappearance of her phobia, the conditional response.

References

Adolphs, R. (2013). The Biology of Fear. *Current Biology, 23*, R79–R93.

Beard C. (2011). Cognitive bias modification for anxiety: current evidence and future directions. *Expert Review of Neurotherapeutics, 11*(2), 299-311. doi:10.1586/ern.10.194.

Crocker, L., Heller, W., Warren, S., O'Hare, A., Infantolio, Z., & Miller, G. (2013). Relationships among cognition, emotion, and motivation: implications for intervention and neuroplasticity in psychopathology. *Front Hum Neurosci., 7*, 261. doi: 10.3389/fnhum.2013.00261

Doctor, R., Kahn, A., & Adamec, C. (2010). *The Encyclopedia of Phobias, Fears, and Anxieties* (3rd Edn). New York, NY: Infobase Publishing.

Foa, E. B., & Kozak, M. (1986). Emotional processing of fear. Exposure to corrective information. *Psychol Bull., 99*, 20-35.

Fryling, M., Johnston, C., & Hayes, L. (2011). Understanding Observational Learning: An Interbehavioral Approach. *Anal Verbal Behav., 27*(1), 191–203.

Galef, B .G. (1988). Imitation in animals: history, definition and interpretation of data from the psychological laboratory. In T. R. Zentall and B. G. Galef (Eds.), *Social Learning: Psychological and Biological Perspectives* (pp. 3-28). Hillsdale, NJ: Erlbaum.

(Henton,W., & Iversen, I. (2012). Classical Conditioning and Operant Conditioning: A Response Pattern Analysis. Berlin, Germany: Springer Science & Business Media.

Hofmann, S. (2008). Cognitive processes during fear acquisition and extinction in animals and humans. *Clin Psychol Rev., 28*(2), 199–210. doi: 10.1016/j.cpr.2007.04.009

Krypotos, A., Effting, M., Kindt, M., & Beckers, T. (2015). Avoidance learning: a review of theoretical models and recent developments. *Front Behav Neurosci., 9*, 189. doi: 10.3389/fnbeh.2015.00189

Lipp, O. V., & Edwards, M. (2002). Effect of instructed extinction on verbal and autonomic indices of Pavlovian learning with fear-relevant conditional stimuli. *Journal of Psychophysiology, 16*, 176–186.

Seligman, L., & Ollendick, T. (2011). Cognitive-Behavioral Therapy for Anxiety Disorders in Youth. *Child and Adolescent Psychiatric Clinics of North America, 20*(2), 217-238. doi:10.1016/j.chc.2011.01.003

YOUR KNOWLEDGE HAS VALUE

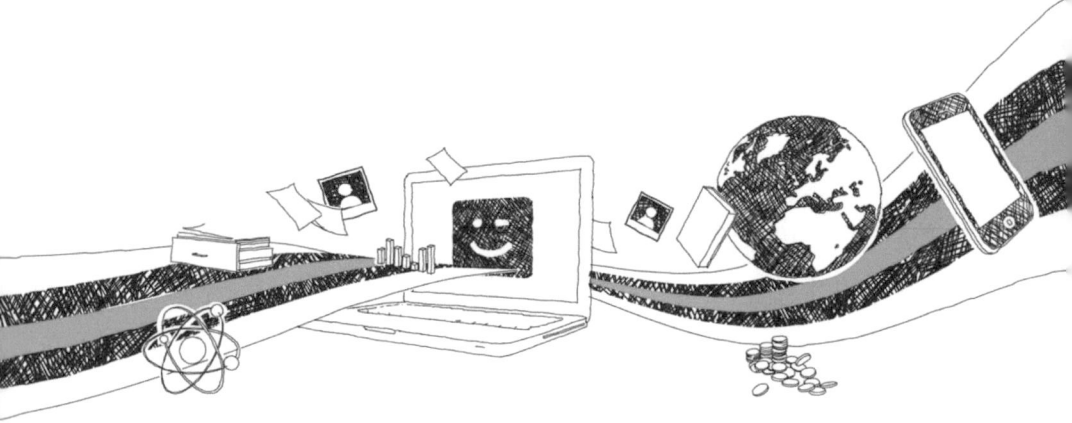

- We will publish your bachelor's and master's thesis, essays and papers

- Your own eBook and book - sold worldwide in all relevant shops

- Earn money with each sale

Upload your text at www.GRIN.com and publish for free

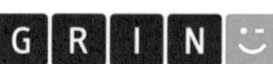